Tanya G. Guleria

Why Immunization Against Covid-19 Causes Heart Attack?

Contents:

Theory of Autoimmunity

I would try to explain this completely new scientific issue quite simple. Let me give you firstly a quick definition of

Immune system:
a diffuse, complex network of interacting cells, cell products and cell forming tissues that protects the body from pathogens another foreign substances,

destroys infected and malignant cells, and removes cellular debris:

Immune system includes the thymus, spleen, lymph nodes and lymph tissue, stem cells, white blood cells, antibodies, and lymphokines.

Human immune system reacts to each protein that consists of more than 20 alfa-amino-acids and different from human proteins. When the proteins enter the gastrointestinal tract most of them are digested and in the form of amino acids can enter the blood stream and be used in the organism as building units.

If the intestinal membrane is not intact, which happens often through chemical or mechanical injuries the foreign protein can enter through the intestine wall into the interstitium and into the lymph stream where it can affect the immune system and cause an immune reaction through producing antibodies against it. It is a normal reaction of the organism to produce antibodies against foreign proteins.

Let us imagine the foreign protein is very similar in structure to a human protein, which can be found on the membrane or in the cytoplasm of a human cell. Then the antibodies of the human organism react falsely to the membrane protein of its own cells and thus induce cellular death through the immune reaction. This assumption may lead to the explanation of all autoimmune diseases and some degenerative diseases like atherosclerosis and diabetes, Alzheimer,

Parkinson, dementia, psychical disorders, autism, obesity and many others.

It is spoken a lot about the connection between irritable bowel syndrome and other diseases. This only proves the theory of autoimmunity, because if someone has irritable bowel syndrome it is more likely ones immune system to react to foreign proteins coming with the food. On one side the erosions in the digestive membrane allow more foreign proteins to enter the interstitium and cause immune reaction. On other side irritable bowel syndrome shows that the person who has this syndrome has already antibodies which attack his own cells.

So is that Pandora`s Box?

Many diseases affect not only humans but also some animal species. This leads to the conclusion that there are similar proteins on the cell membranes and in the cytoplasm in humans and animals. Digesting similar to our proteins may lead to an autoimmune reaction against our proteins and degeneration of some tissues like blood endothelium, respiratory endothelium cells, Langerhans cells of the pancreas, the cells of the nephrons, or even the death or destruction of brain cells, causing great number of diseases.

An Example for the autoimmune theory is Diabetes Mellitus Type 1

Diabetes mellitus type 1 has long been known medical disease. But lethality of diabetes begins only when people begin to therapy it. Why?

It has long been known that diabetes type 1 is caused by an immune response to beta cells of the islets of Langerhans (of the same which go on vacation).

1. It is known that the immune system responds only to proteins, i.e., Why not to the protein of insulin?

2. It is known that porcine insulin differs by only 2 amino acids from human. I.e. why not exogenously induced immune response (e.g. alimentarian autoimmune reaction)? The porcine insulin in the food gets into the gastro-intestinal tract, thence through erosions of the gastrointestinal tract gets into the lymphatic system, where antibodies against it are built. These antibodies react against porcine insulin and against human insulin (because they are common in structure). Thus they destroy the beta-cells of the islets of Langerhans by an immune reaction type B. It leads to the conclusion that Type 1 diabetes is caused by autoimmunity against insulin.

In conclusion: bovine and porcine insulin are too common with human insulin. They are foreign protein molecules and cause immune reaction, the antibodies built against them react also to human insulin and cause the destruction of Beta-cells in pancreas, inducing diabetes type I.

Another Example of the Logic of the Autoimmune Theory is Diabetes Mellitus Type II

Bovine and porcine receptors to insulin are also common with human receptors. Consuming big amounts of them, found in the muscle tissue of animals, causes the production of human antibodies against them. These antibodies connect themselves with human insulin receptors in human organism. That causes insulin resistance in human tissues. On back-forth connection mechanism this causes increasing of insulin levels in blood. This causes constant hunger and increasing of food consumption, thus obesity and metabolic syndrome. In this vicious circle soon the capacity of human Langerhans cells to produce insulin is exhausted and this leads to diabetes type II.

Obesity is often associated with the development of insulin resistance. According to the popular way to overcome insulin resistance, those affected should consume meat and meat products and avoid carbohydrates that are rich in plants. However, this is completely wrong. According to autoimmune theory, insulin resistance and obesity are caused by eating meat with the food. Through food in meat in the GIT enter a lot of animal insulin receptors (because muscle tissue is rich with them) they pass through the intestinal wall into the interstitium and in the lymph stream. These foreign proteins elicit an immune response and the production of antibodies that mistakenly respond to the human insulin receptors, causing insulin resistance and subsequent obesity and diabetes type 2. Therefore, the most appropriate treatment for obesity and diabetes is the exclusion of animal products of food.

Consumption of Poultry and Bird Products may have a Connection with Chronical Respiratory and Blood Vessel Diseases

Influenza virus affects different animal species like humans, birds and pigs. That means that the receptor which lets the influenza virus into the respiratory and blood vessel cells is common in these species. This receptor consumed with food gets into gastro-intestinal tract and into the lymphatic system, antibodies against it are built and they react against it and falsely against human respiratory and blood vessel cells which have a common in structure receptor. So a chronic autoimmune disease is caused such as bronchial asthma, COPD, emphysema, autoimmune blood vessel deceases and perhaps also atherosclerosis, thus brain strokes, myocardial infarction and others.

It is largely spoken about the connection between cholesterol and atherosclerosis. There are two sources of cholesterol in blood: exogenous and endogenous. The exogenous or alimentary is 20% of all, and endogenous source is 80%. The endogenous is a result of the own organism's production in connection with the building and demolition of cell membrane. In my opinion the high levels of cholesterol in blood is not the reason for atherosclerosis, but a result from it. By atherosclerosis by an autoimmune mechanism is demolished the endothelium membrane, and this leads to high cholesterol blood levels. The autoimmune demolition of endothelium membranes leads to accumulation of binding tissue and into it incorporate fat , because of its high level in blood, as a result from the demolition of cell membranes by autoimmunity. Therefore not cholesterol in food but consumption of meat leads to atherosclerosis.

Empirically is proven that vegetarians have lower levels of cholesterol and atherosclerosis. Why? In fact vegetables contain almost the same level of cholesterol as meat, because it is a part of their cell membrane. Usually medical doctors prohibit the consumption of pork and bird skin, because they are oilier. But according to the autoimmune theory it is not enough, because meat inclusive bird and eggs contain not only cholesterol, but also the so called influenza receptor. It is well known in microbiology that influenza virus develops wonderfully on the egg membrane, influenza virus affects also birds. The receptor for influenza virus in birds and eggs membrane has a very similar analogue in human respiratory and blood vessel cells. That is the reason why we all (humans and birds) get sick with influenza. The antibodies which our immune system builds against the bird receptor, which is found in bird's meat, react to the human influenza receptor and cause respiratory and blood vessels deceases such as atherosclerosis resulting in peripheral vascular diseases, coronary vascular diseases and heart attacks and ischemic brain strokes.

15

Laboratory tests prove that not only so called autoimmune diseases such as lupus erythematosus, rheumatoid arthritis, Morbus Bechtereff, thyroiditis of Hashimoto, Basedoff disease contain an element of inflammation, but also degenerative diseases like atherosclerosis, diabetes, obesity, psychical disorders such as autism, psychoses, dementia, Parkinson syndrome, myasthenia gravis and many others. But until now no one has explained why. We all thought that cholesterol damages the blood vessel like a stone. It accumulates in the blood vessel interstitium and causes immune reaction and inflammation. But this idea does not make sense at all, does it?

Cholesterol is a building part of cell, so how could it damage the blood vessel? It is like hitting the vessel with a dilution of sugar or oil at a slow speed and expecting it would be damaged.

It is like aiming at rabbits with carrots. It could be deadly, isn't it?

The truth is the organism acquires high levels of cholesterol as a result from higher cell membrane demolition trough the autoimmune reaction caused by the antibodies built against the receptor proteins in meat. In the vessel accumulates binding tissue after the immune reaction and it binds cholesterol in its interstitium, thus causing atherosclerosis in all of its forms.

So in conclusion atherosclerosis is caused by autoimmune reaction. It is inflammatory reaction and high level of cholesterol is a result not a purpose for it.

In fact statin therapy of high level of cholesterol is completely purposeless, because it is like fighting with a biochemical substance which is not the reason for atherosclerosis, but a result from it. And statins have a lot of side effects. You can check it by yourselves.

Angiotensin converting enzyme 2

Angiotensin converting enzyme 2, or ACE2, is an exopeptidase expressed primarily by vascular endothelial cells in the heart and kidneys, but also in respiratory epithelia[1] and in the gastrointestinal tract. It is the target of several coronaviruses, including SARS-CoV and SARS-CoV-2.

2 Biochemistry

ACE2 is a transmembrane metallocarboxypeptidase composed of 805 amino acids. Zinc and chloride ions act as cofactors. The extracellular region consists of two domains, a zinc metallopeptidase domain and a C-terminal collectrin homology domain. The enzyme exhibits homology to angiotensin converting enzyme (ACE).

ACE2 is encoded by the ACE2 gene on the X chromosome (gene locus Xp22.2). In addition to being expressed as a transmembrane protein, a soluble form exists in serum.

3 Function

ACE2 cleaves angiotensin II into angiotensin (1-7), which has anti-inflammatory and lung protective effects via MAS and AT2 receptors.

4 Clinical

4.1 Infectiology

ACE2 serves as a major entry point for some coronaviruses. The pathogens bind to the enzyme with their spike proteins and enter the host cell by subsequent fusion.[2] ACE2 expression increases from the pharynx to the alveoli. In addition, SARS-CoV-2 is thought to have a higher affinity for ACE2 than SARS-CoV. This would explain more rapid and effective viral transmission in the COVID-19 pandemic.

Patients taking drugs that increase the expression of ACE2 - for example, ACE inhibitors or sartans, may be at higher risk of infection and should be switched to calcium antagonists, according to some authors.[3][4] In contrast, the relevant professional societies see no need for action at this time (4/2020).[5][6]

4.2 Pharmacology

Human recombinant ACE2 (APN01) is an experimental therapeutic approach being tested in acute respiratory distress syndrome (ARDS) and pulmonary hypertension.[7] Furthermore, it is currently (2020) being tested for the treatment of COVID-19.[8][9]

5 Sources

1. Hong Peng Jia et al. ACE2 Receptor Expression and Severe Acute Respiratory Syndrome Coronavirus Infection Depend on Differentiation of Human Airway Epithelia, J Virol. 2005 Dec; 79(23): 14614-14621, retrieved 2020 Mar 27.

2. Kuba K et al. A crucial role of angiotensin converting enzyme 2 (ACE2) in SARS

coronavirus-induced lung injury, Nat Med. 2005 Aug;11(8):875-9. epub 2005 Jul 10, retrieved 2020 Mar 30.

3. Zheng Y et al. COVID-19 and the cardiovascular system, Nat Rev Cardiol (2020), retrieved 30 Mar 2020.

4. Fang, L. et al. Are patients with hypertension and diabetes mellitus at increased risk for COVID-19 infection?, The Lancet, March 2020, retrieved 27/03/2020.

5. ESC Position Statement of the ESC Council on Hypertension on ACE Inhibitors and Angiotensin Receptor Blockers, retrieved March 27, 2020.

6. The Renal Association, UK position statement for patients: novel corona virus infection and the use of blood pressure medications. retrieved 03/27/2020.

7. Zhang H, Baker A Recombinant human ACE2: acing out angiotensin II in ARDS

therapy, Crit Care. 2017 Dec 13;21(1):305, retrieved 2020 Mar 30.

8. Zhang H et al. Angiotensin-converting enzyme 2 (ACE2) as a SARS-CoV-2 receptor: molecular mechanisms and potential therapeutic target, Intensive Care Med. 2020 Apr;46(4):586-590, retrieved 2020 Mar 30.

9. clinicaltrials.gov APN01, retrieved 03/30/2020.

CoViD-19 and ACE inhibitors

The disease is often moderate or even asymptomatic. However, severe courses can occur, usually manifesting as pneumonia. In some of the seriously ill patients, severe cardiovascular damage is also observed.

For people with heart disease, the disease - which is caused by the SARS-CoV-2 virus - thus appears to be particularly dangerous.

Angiotensin-converting enzyme 2 (ACE2) plays a major role in the body's water balance. ACE inhibitors lower blood pressure and reduce afterload - which also makes them very useful in treating heart failure disease.

ACE2 are particularly abundant in the heart and lungs. Currently, attention is focused on this enzyme because ACE2 has been identified as a functional receptor for the coronaviruses SARS-CoV and SARS-CoV-2.

It appears that the amount of ACE2 increases by taking ACE2 inhibitors in response. Thus, the body responds to inhibition of these receptors by increasing potential docking sites.

It has not yet been proven whether this mechanism promotes or exacerbates the disease!

Up-regulating ACE2 may also have benefits: The enzyme protects the heart and vasculature by cleaving angiotensin II-which promotes hypertension, edema, and tissue damage-and thereby inactivating it.

In SARS-CoV infection, ACE2 is downregulated as an antiviral protective measure: Angiotensin II can then promote severe tissue damage during infection. ACE inhibitors and sartans could therefore be helpful because they slow down angiotensin II formation or block the corresponding receptor, respectively ...

It is a fact that special attention is paid to patients with underlying cardiovascular disease in connection with covid-19 disease. Recently, experts from the U.S. Cardiac Society (ACC) considered the viral epidemic from a cardiology perspective in an official letter of recommendation. The society makes nine recommendations for managing the coronavirus epidemic.

The experts recommend that "consistent use of guideline-based therapy with plaque-stabilizing agents (statins, beta blockers, ACE inhibitors, ASS) provides additional protection for cardiac patients, and such treatment should be tailored to individual patients." Accordingly, these experts do not currently consider ACE inhibitors to be critical.

That this is a preliminary assessment is reflected in point 9 of the recommendation: here, the experts point out that little is currently known about coronavirus and physicians should be prepared for new recommendations as more information becomes available.

Source: www.pharmazeutische-zeitung.de/

Why Immunization Against Covid-19 Causes Heart Attack?

The so called protective function of the vaccine against Covid-19 is based on the fact that the Spyke protein of Covid-19 coming into contact with our immune system causes the production of antibodies which react with this spyke protein.

The human macrophage incorporates this spyke protein on its cell membrane and presents it to the B-cells which produce antibodies against it.

Of course we should not forget that this spyke protein has a structure which responds to the ACE-2 receptor. This means that those Macrophages could connect themselves directly with the corresponding ACE-2 receptor through the spyke protein which is expressed on their cell membrane, causing a quick non-specific immune reaction directly against vascular endothelial cells in the heart and kidneys, but also in respiratory epithelia and in the gastrointestinal tract. Perhaps this is the cause of the very quick and sharpened reaction of many people to the vaccine against Covid-19 which is often connected with later heart disease.

In our practice as general practitioners we often speak to people which connect the first symptoms of myocardial infarction with the application of the Covid-19 vaccine of any type.

Connecting macrophages with vascular endothelial cells causes an inflammation of the coronary vessels, resulting as a vasculitis or myocardial infarction

Of course we have the same result also if we present the Covid-19 directly as an infection with the virus, because its spyke protein is also an important part of the inducing of the immune response to its existence.

The spyke protein expressed on the macrophage cell membrane causes the production of antibodies by the B-cells. Those antibodies connect with it, but we should not forget that they could connect to ACE-inhibitors, which are used in the therapy of hypertension, thus lowering their effects. Perhaps this is one of the reasons why heart patients with ACE-inhibitors in their therapy tend to react worse to Covid-19 infection, but also do not profit a lot by the vaccine.

The result of the vaccine against Covid-19, or the infection cause by it induces the production of antibodies which react against ACE-inhibitors thus neutralizing their effect.

Of course this is only the molecular point of view.

The Implication of antibodies against the ACE-2 receptor which block the connection of Covid-19 with it may also be dangerous, because those foreign antibodies could be incorporated in the macrophage membrane, causing clustering of macrophages which have the spike protein on their cell membrane with macrophages which contain the corresponding structure of the foreign antibodies. Again is induced a severe autoimmune inflammation of the coronary vessel.

Antibodies which connect with the foreign antibodies against ACE2 Receptors also reduce the function of ACE-inhibitors causing often the increase of arterial hypertonia.

Conclusion

In conclusion I must say that Covid-19 infection is a very complex disease which induces a cascade of immune and autoimmune reactions and we could use it as a base point of the proof of the theory of autoimmunity.

Firstly it is proven that Covid-19 connects to a receptor which is known to have a connection with the regulation of high blood pressure and a lot of other functions of the organism as it is proven to exist in many organs and tissues as vascular endothelial cells in the heart and kidneys, but also in respiratory epithelia and in the gastrointestinal tract.

The members of the family *Coronaviridae*, a monophyletic cluster in the order *Nidovirales*, are enveloped, positive stranded RNA viruses of three classes of vertebrates: mammals (corona -and toroviruses), birds (coronaviruses) and fish (bafiniviruses). Virions are spherical, 120–160 nm across (*Coronavirinae*), bacilliform, 170–200×75–88 nm (*Bafinivirus*) or found as a mixture of both, with bacilliform particles characteristically bent into crescents (*Torovirus*). The particles are typically decorated with large, club- or petal-shaped surface projections (the "peplomers" or "spikes"), which in electron micrographs of spherical particles create an image reminiscent of the solar corona. This inspired the name of the "true" coronaviruses (now grouped in the subfamily *Coronavirinae*), which was later adopted for the whole family. Nucleocapsids are helical and can be released from the virion by treatment with detergents. Whereas the coronavirus nucleocapsid appears to be loosely-wound, those of the *Torovirinae* are distinctively tubular. In terms of genome size and genetic complexity, the *Coronaviridae* are the largest RNA viruses identified so far, rivaled only by the okaviruses, large nidoviruses of invertebrates assigned to the

31

family *Roniviridae*. Replication has been studied in detail only for coronaviruses, but the limited data available for toro- and bafiniviruses suggest that the latter viruses use essentially similar strategies. Virions attach to dedicated host cell surface receptors via their spikes and release their genome into the target cell via fusion of the viral envelope with the plasma membrane and/or the limiting membrane of an endocytic vesicle. The entire replication cycle takes place in the cytoplasm and involves the production of full-length and subgenome-sized (sg) minus-strand RNA intermediates with the viral genome serving both as mRNA for the replicase polyproteins and as a template for minus-strand synthesis. RNA synthesis is catalyzed by an as yet poorly characterized replication–transcription complex, composed of viral and host proteins and associated (at least in coronaviruses) with an interconnected network of modified intracellular membranes and double-membrane vesicles that are presumably endoplasmic reticulum (ER)-derived.

The conclusion is that Corona viruses are wide spread in nature, affect animals and humans. They enter the cells through a receptor ACE 2 which is found on endothelial cells of blood vessels, which is amongst all also responsible for regulating blood pressure.

So if we consume those animals our immune system gets in contact with those receptors which are big protein molecules and our immune system produces antibodies against those receptors.

Those antibodies may have an important part of inducing an autoimmune reaction against the endothelial cells thus causing atherosclerosis, resulting as a myocardial infarction, periphery vessels atherosclerosis, brain strokes and further.

ACE2 receptors are also found in kidneys and we all know that the damage of the kidney function causes hypertension. So the damage of kidney ACE receptors may be the cause of arterial hypertension and kidney failure. The theme of arterial hypertension I presented in my book "New View on Antihypertensive Therapy"

ACE receptors are found in respiratory epithelium so antibodies against it may cause also asthma and COPD by non-smokers. This theme I mentioned in my first book "Theory of autoimmunity" and perhaps would be the theme of my next book.

Nevertheless the main theme of this book is Covid-19 Infection and the effects of the vaccine against Covid-19 I cannot deny the connection with my first book which is the "Theory of Autoimmunity". All conclusions are based on this theory which is a very ambitious project to explain most important diseases in our society.

The theory of autoimmunity is the most important project to which I have dedicated the studies of all my life, reading, analyzing and connecting a lot of medical articles.

The problem of modern medicine is that it is so concentrated in cells, molecules and chemical substances that it should be divided in different specialties in order to cover the expanding medical knowledge of molecules, cells and chemical substances. This is the reason why we forget to summon our knowledge into an all including "theory of everything".

Theory of autoimmunity does not imply to explain "everything", but it is very logical and systematic and this is what we lack in official medicine: logic and system.

I hope you enjoyed reading this book and I hope of new encounter.

www.ingramcontent.com/pod-product-compliance
Lightning Source LLC
Chambersburg PA
CBHW072239230526
45466CB00025B/2167